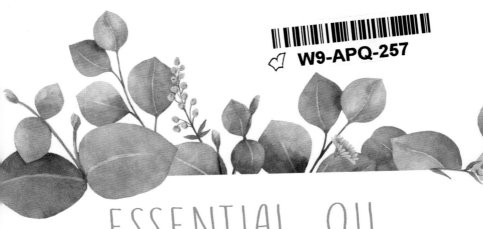

ESSENTIAL OIL

make & takes

OVER 60 DIY PROJECTS AND RECIPES FOR THE PERFECT CLASS

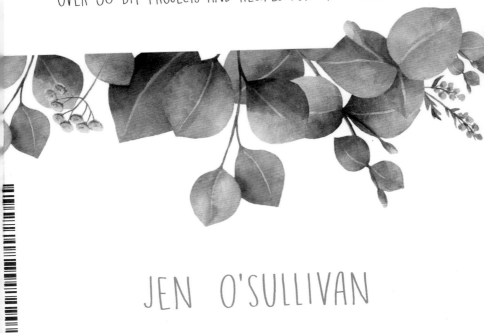

JEN O'SULLIVAN

ESSENTIAL OIL MAKE & TAKES *by Jen O'Sullivan*

Copyright ©2017 by Jen O'Sullivan
www.31oils.com

Book Designed by 31 Oils
Cover Art by Elena Medvedeva
Edited by Tina Bosse

ISBN: 978-1545411636

Printed in the United States of America

May, 2017

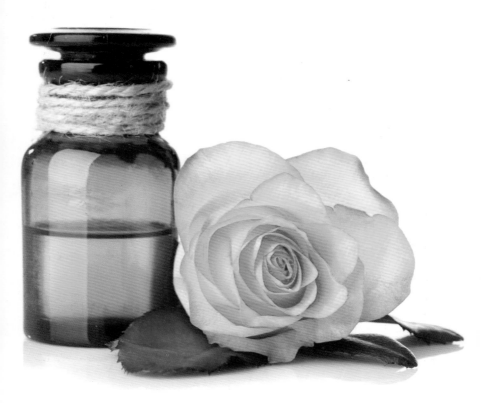

CONTENTS

4 HOW TO HOST A CLASS

6 THE RECIPES

6 Baby Bottom Paste

6 Baby Gum Soothing Serum

7 Baby Scalp Scrub & Serum

8 Bath Salts

9 Bath Soak (Oatmeal)

9 Bikini Line Serum

10 Body Sugar Scrub

11 Body Wash

11 Bubble Bath

12 Car Vent Diffuser

13 Cool-Down Spray

13 Critter Spray

14 Face Cleanser

15 Face Exfoliator

16 Eye Serum

16 Face Serum (All Skin Types)

17 Face Serum (Blemish Support)

17 Face Toner Spray

18 Fingernail Support

18 Fizzies (Bath Bombs)

19 Fragrance

20 Hand Lotion

21 Hand Soap (Foaming)

21 Hand Scrubbing Balls

22 Hair Conditioning Rinse

22 Hair Deep Cleanser

23 Hair Deep Conditioner

24 Hair Detangling Spray

24 Hair Detangling Spray (Easy)

25 Hair Dry Shampoo

26 Hair Follicle Spray

27 Hair Serum

27 Hair Shampoo

28 Hair Split End Spray

Hair Shine Spray 28

Heel and Foot Cream 29

Home: Candles 30

Home: Degreaser 31

Home: Drawer Sachets 31

Home: Room Freshener 32

Home: Window Cleaner 32

Hydrosol 33

Lip Balm 34

Lip Scrub 34

Lucy Libido's Skinamint 35

Makeup Removing Pads 35

Manly Aftershave 36

Manly Beard Balm 36

Manly Beard Oil 37

Manly Muscle Support 37

Mouthwash 38

Nipple Butter 39

Potty-pourri Spray 39

Rollerballs 40

Scalp Serum Mask 41

Scalp Spray 41

Sunscreen 42

Toenail Support 43

Tooth Polish 43

Underarm Support 44

Underarm Support (Easy) 44

Whipped Body Butter 45

FINAL THOUGHTS 46

RESOURCES 49

EQUIPMENT LIST 49

SUPPLY LIST 49

INGREDIENT LIST 50

ADDITIONAL EDUCATION 52

AUTHOR BIOGRAPHY 53

HOW TO HOST A MAKE & TAKE CLASS

Hosting a Make & Take Essential Oil party can be exciting and fun, yet completely overwhelming and very hard on your pocketbook. It is easy to go crazy making what we think will "wow" our guests by Martha-ing the party to death! You know the drill- clean the house top to bottom, create the most delicious oil-infused food, goodies, and treats, have Lavender Spa Lemonade... and forget about dull make and take items - you go all out by coming up with 6 amazing DIY Make & Take stations all throughout your kitchen, dining room, and living room. You even have a great decorating station, complete with the cutest DIY labels, pens, and washi tape. You make plans to have your husband and kids all go to a movie to have the whole house to yourself. The guests arrive to the most fun they have had at an in-home party that they can remember. You socialize and laugh hysterically, make great oily projects, decorate them all to the nines, and everyone leaves with amazing products to try... and NO ONE buys a kit!

The sad reality is that this happens more often than not. Make & Takes, while very fun, are not IPAs (Income Producing Activities). There are two types of people who come to a Make & Take: current customers and potential customers. Strategically invite so you know which type of Make & Take party to throw. For ease of describing the parties, the Make & Take parties for newbies who are not yet customers will be referred to as" Make & Take 101." For current customers, these parties will be referred to as "Make & Take 102." The concept is to create a fun class for new people as an Oil 101 combined with an easy introduction Make & Take that only uses oils in the Premium Starter Kit (PSK). Make it super simple and easy. Do not overdo it. Resist the urge! For your current customers, you would also make it simple, but create a customer appreciation class where you teach a more advanced project and you introduce oils outside the PSK.

This book contains some of the most loved Make & Take projects and will help you determine which type of party they are best suited for. You will also notice the projects are made with oils from the PSK, or there will be a line item that suggests which PSK oil to use as an alternative. All item sizes are based on personal use. It is suggested you use the smallest size available. For instance, instead of using a 15mL dropper bottle, cut the recipe in thirds and use a 5mL dropper, or even smaller by using a 2mL dropper bottle. Make sure the cost for all items totals less than $3 each with all supplies. For the Make & Take 102, your customers would bring their own oils and you would introduce new oils for them to smell (but not use). Teach them how to add the new oils after class. If you would rather allow them to use your oils, it is very important that you make smaller sample-size batches and charge accordingly. Msking full-size eye serums for everyone will get very expensive, and the goal is to have them purchase their own oils to make the project again after class. Enjoy making all the fun items in this book!

The following are instructions on how to host a successful Make & Take class that is also an Oil 101 Class. You can find more details on information in the book "Essentially Driven: Young Living Essential Oils® Business Handbook."

• Invite 4 times as many people as you would like to attend.
• Personally invite each person 1-2 weeks before the event. Do not send out a group email or e-vite. A personal phone call, text message, or email is fine depending on the person.
　Sample invite: Hi Amy! Several of us ladies are getting together at my place next
　week on (date and time) to make candles and to chat about essential oils. Can you
　join us? I love candles but hate the ones form the store because they give me such a

headache. We are going to make chemical free candles that are super easy. Let me know if you can make it so I can order the right amount of supplies!

• If the person says they can come, leave out some information so you can have multiple connection points as reminders.

Example connection points:

~4 days before, ask if they have any friends they would like to bring so you can have enough supplies for the group project.

~2 days before, give them your address.

~1 day before, share that you are very excited about the party and ask them what their favorite color is (you can use this info to pick up some ribbon for the make and take for them to personalize it).

~Day of, let them know your door will be unlocked and to come on in.

1. Get the class started with a DIY Make & Take project. This will allow guests who arrive late to not miss the important EO things. Use one of the Oil 101 projects in this book.

2. After the project is complete, either continue in the room you are in, or gather your guests to the main presentation room. Welcome your guests again and share a little about you and why you got into oils. Tell a short 3-5 minute testimonial about how oils have changed and enhanced your life and tie it into the Make & Take item you just made.

3. Briefly introduce the starter kit. Share the price up front: both retail and wholesale.

4. Go over the basics of essential oils in under 60 seconds.

Sample: Essential oils are the life-force of plants. They help the plant to regulate itself and add health and overall wellness. These oils can work in much the same way for us. There are three ways to use essential oils: aromatic, topical, and internal. It takes 20 minutes for essential oils to reach every cell in your body from the time you apply them. There are around 100 trillion cells in our bodies, and one drop of essential oil contains orer 40 million trillion molecules! This menas every single cell in our body, in 20 minutes, is covered by 40,000 essential oil molecules.

5. Go over each oil in the Premium Starter Kit and pass it around as you discuss it so everyone can smell it. This is the best time to tell your stories.

6. Share why Young Living is different from all other brands. Cover the Seed to Seal® process. This is a great time to do a smell test using 3 oils (optional). Use peppermint from Young Living and two other companies, such as a major competitor and one that you can buy in a grocery store. All of them should be covered up so you do not disclose who the other brands are. This becomes a wonderful opportunity to share the difference between how oils are processed and why the smell can help you know the difference. Share the "Quality Chart" found in "Essentially Driven." Young Living oils always smell more earthy, while the others will have a sweeter smell.

7. Go over what is in the kit, the retail price at $325, and then the wholesale price at $160.

8. Ask happily and in a heartfelt way if anyone would like to buy a kit, host a party, or join your team! Share briefly what the business has done for you and how you would love to help them host their first party. Then tell them, "First things first, I want you to fall head over heels in love with your oils, so let's order your kit!" Ask for the sale. Don't just wrap it up and say goodnight. Don't peter out with a Q&A session. Get oils into their home!

9. End on time and don't forget to laugh and have fun. Do not do anything over-produced at parties. Simple, pretty, and fun is best! Don't go crazy stressing yourself out about it. Think of it like a fun girls' night out. The more over the top you make your classes, the harder it will be for others to envision themselves doing it. You want people to say, "Wow, I could totally do this!"

10. For those who did not buy a kit, find out why and then follow up. Be friendly, yet persistent. Continue to share your love and passion for the oils and why you know they will love them too!

11. Do it again and again and again! Practice makes perfect, and while classses do not need to be perfect, your nerves will be more settled the more you teach.

BABY BOTTOM PASTE

Ingredients:
- 4 ounce Glass Jar
- 4 tablespoons Shea Butter
- 2 tablespoons Zinc Oxide Powder
- 1 tablespoon Jojoba Oil
- 2 tableapoons Aloe Vera Gel
- 10 drops of Gentle Baby® Essential Oil
- PSK Alternative: 5 drops each Lavender and Frankincense

DIY Directions: In a double boiler, melt shea butter until just melted. Turn off burner and add Jojoba oil, Aloe Vera Gel, and essential oils and blend well. Slowly stir in Zinc Oxide Powder, a small amount at a time, until it is fully blended. Pour lotion into jar and seal tightly to let cool.

> *Note: Zinc Oxide powder is very fome. Wear gloves and do not allow any to get into your lungs. Do not have small children in the room when working with the powder form of Zinc Oxide. While Zinc Oxide is a natural ingredient and is non-toxic, it should not be inhaled.*

Directions for Use: Apply to baby's bottom as needed during a diaper change.

Party Type: Make & Take 102

BABY GUM SOOTHING SERUM

Ingredients:
- 5mL Dropper Bottle
- Jojoba Oil
- 5 drops each Clove and Lavender essential oils
- PSK Alternative: 5 drops each Lavender and Thieves®

DIY Directions: Combine essential oils in the dropper bottle and swirl to blend. Top off with Jojoba carrier oil.

Directions for Use: Apply to baby's gums as needed.

Party Type: Make & Take 101

BABY SCALP SCRUB & SERUM

Ingredients for scalp scrub:
- 2 ounce Glass Jar
- 2 tablespoons Jojoba Oil
- 1 tablespoon Coconut Oil (Alternative: Jojoba Oil)
- 1-2 tablespoons Baking Soda
- 5 drops Gentle Baby® Essential Oil
- PSK Alternative: 3 drops each Lavender and Frankincense

DIY Directions: Combine all ingredients and blend well.

Ingredients for Scalp Serum
- 15mL Dropper Bottle
- 1 tablespoon Jojoba Oil
- 3 drops each Lavender and Frankincense

DIY Directions: Combine essential oils in the dropper bottle and swirl to blend. Top off with Jojoba oil and swirl to blend.

Directions for Use: Apply Scalp Scrub to baby's scalp 2 times daily in a circular motion. Use a warm microfiber cloth to gently rinse off. Apply 2-3 drops of the Scalp Serum directly after rubbing off scrub.

Party Type: Make & Take 102

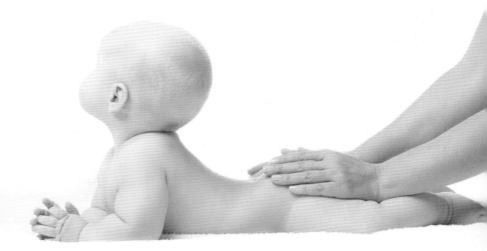

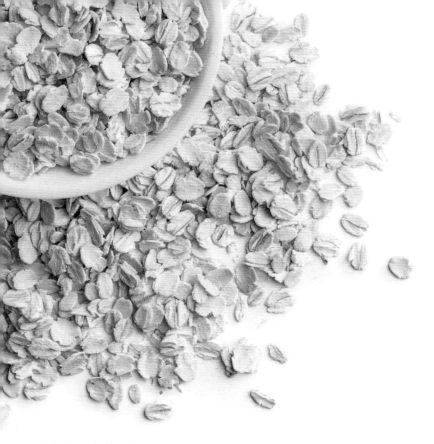

BATH SALTS

Ingredients:
- 8 ounce Mason Jar
- 1 ¾ cups Epsom Salt
- ¼ cup Baking Soda
- 8-10 drops of Lavender or Stress Away™ Essential Oil

DIY Directions: Combine salt and Baking Soda in jar, add essential oils, place lid on tightly, and shake to disperse.

Directions for Use: Pour entire contents into a warm bath and enjoy!

Party Type: Make & Take 101

BATH SOAK (OATMEAL)

Ingredients :
- 8 ounce Glass Jar
- 1 cup Epsom Salt
- 1 cup Gluten Free Oats (Quick Oats)
- ½ cup Baking Soda
- 15 drops Peace & Calming™ Essential Oil
- PSK Alternative Essential Oils: Lavender or Stress Away™

DIY Directions : Grind Oats and Epsom Salt in a coffee grinder until it is a fine texture. Add Baking Soda and essential oils. Blend well and place into glass jar.

Directions for Use : Pour 1 cup into a hot bath and soak for 30 minutes.

Party Type : Make & Take 101

BIKINI LINE SERUM

Ingredients :
- 15mL Dropper Bottle
- Grapeseed Oil
- 30 drops Grapefruit or Melrose™ Essential Oil
- PSK Alternative Essential Oils: Lemon or Purification®

DIY Directions : Combine Grapeseed oil and Grapefruit (or Lemon) for winter and Melrose™ (or Purification®) for summer. Fasten on the cap, then swirl the bottle to blend well.

Directions for Use : Apply a dime-size amount over shaved areas right after you towel off from the shower.

Party Type : Make & Take 101

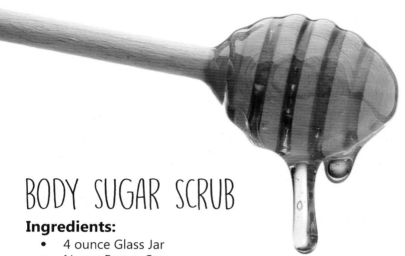

BODY SUGAR SCRUB

Ingredients:

- 4 ounce Glass Jar
- ¼ cup Brown Sugar
- ¼ cup Raw Cane Sugar
- 2 tablespoons Grapeseed oil
- 2 tablespoons Organic Honey (optional)
- Melted Raw Coconut Oil to desired consistency (Alternative: Grapeseed or Jojoba oil)
- 10-15 drops Lemon Essential Oil

DIY Directions: Combine all ingredients in a bowl and blend to a wet sand consistency. It should not be crumbly, but more soupy in texture. Scoop into jar and place lid on tightly. Do not fill to the top or the oils will seep out.

Directions for Use: Scoop out a handful and scrub over freshly-washed body in the shower. Rinse off with warm water and towel dry for supple soft skin!

Party Type: Make & Take 101

BODY WASH

Ingredients:
- 8 ounce Glass Bottle or Foaming Soap Dispenser
- ½ cup Liquid Castile Soap
- 4 tablespoons Vegetable Glycerin
- 3 tablespoons Sweet Almond Oil
- 10 drops each Peppermint, Lavender, and Lemon Essential Oils

DIY Directions: Combine all essential oils in bottle and swirl to blend. Add Vegetable Glycerin and Sweet Almond oil and swirl to blend. Add Castile soap and shake well to fully blend.
> *Note: Alternative for use as a Foaming Body Wash: fill foaming soap container to ¼ full. Top off with distilled water and shake to blend.*

Directions for Use: Use in the shower with a loofah or washcloth.

Party Type: Make & Take 101

BUBBLE BATH

Ingredients:
- 4 ounce Glass Bottle
- ½ cup Liquid Castile Soap (Natural Way Organics)
- ¼ cup Vegetable Glycerin
- 2 tablespoons White Granulated Sugar
- 1 Egg White (optional for larger bubbles)
- 10 drops Tangerine Essential Oil
- PSK Alternative Essential Oils: Lavender or Stress Away™

DIY Directions: Combine all ingredients and shake to blend.

Directions for Use: Pour half of contents under running bath water. Place remaining contents in refrigerator to be used within a week.
> *Note: Natural bubble bath recipes generally do not work. I have tried too many to count and all have failed. This is the best one I have come up with. The trick is using the correct type of Castile soap. You need to use one that is made out of Saponified Coconut oil. Natural Way Organics is a good one. The bubbles will not compare to store-bought bubble bath but you will have fun tor a minute or two and won't have to deal with all the nasty chemicals in the store-bought ones .*

Party Type: Make & Take 102

CAR VENT DIFFUSER

Ingredients:

- 1 Clothespin
- Wood Glue
- Raw Wood or Cork Embellishments
- 5 drops Peppermint or Purification® Essential Oil

DIY Directions: Glue on embellishments to your liking. Allow to fully dry.

Directions for Use: Apply essential oil to cork or raw wood and click clothespin onto air vent. Run air as normal based on desired temperature. This can also work well for hotel rooms. Clip onto air conditioner outflow vent and run air to freshen the room.

Party Type: Make & Take 101

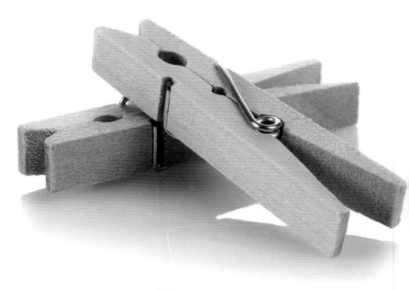

COOL-DOWN SPRAY

Ingredients:
- 2 ounce Glass Spray Bottle
- 1 ounce Distilled Water
- 1 ounce Witch Hazel
- 20 drops Peppermint Essential Oil

DIY Directions: Combine the essential oil and Witch Hazel in the bottle and swirl to blend. Top off with distilled water and swirl to blend.

Directions for Use: Spray liberally on skin to cool down as needed. For men, this works great to spray across the shoulders and back. For women, during menopause, spray anywhere as needed. Do not spray in eyes. If you want to spray on the face, sight down, close eyes tightly, mist over face, and keep eyes closed until mist dries completely.

Party Type: Make & Take 101

CRITTER SPRAY

Ingredients:
- 2 ounce Spray Bottle
- Distilled Water
- Witch Hazel
- 1 tablespoon Jojoba Oil
- 100 drops (yes, 100 drops)Purification® Essential Oil

DIY Directions: Combine the essential oil and Jojoba oil in the dropper bottle and swirl to blend. Add Witch Hazel to half full and swirl to blend. Top off with distilled water and swirl again.

Directions for Use: Spray liberally on exposed skin every 1-2 hours when outdoors.

Party Type: Make & Take 102

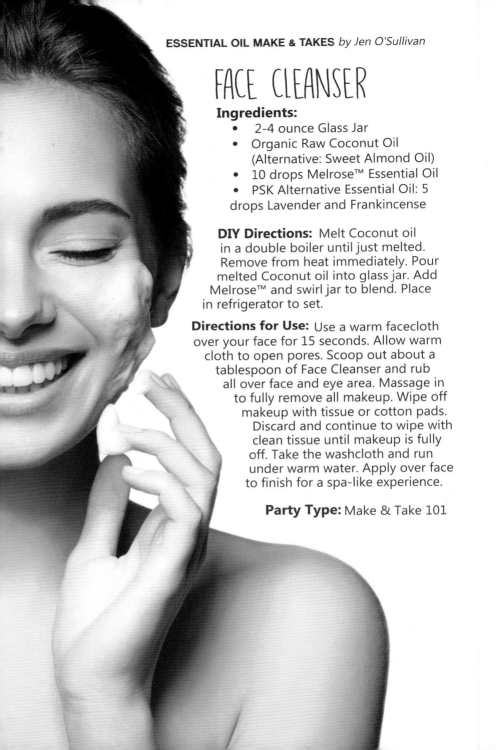

FACE CLEANSER

Ingredients:
- 2-4 ounce Glass Jar
- Organic Raw Coconut Oil (Alternative: Sweet Almond Oil)
- 10 drops Melrose™ Essential Oil
- PSK Alternative Essential Oil: 5 drops Lavender and Frankincense

DIY Directions: Melt Coconut oil in a double boiler until just melted. Remove from heat immediately. Pour melted Coconut oil into glass jar. Add Melrose™ and swirl jar to blend. Place in refrigerator to set.

Directions for Use: Use a warm facecloth over your face for 15 seconds. Allow warm cloth to open pores. Scoop out about a tablespoon of Face Cleanser and rub all over face and eye area. Massage in to fully remove all makeup. Wipe off makeup with tissue or cotton pads. Discard and continue to wipe with clean tissue until makeup is fully off. Take the washcloth and run under warm water. Apply over face to finish for a spa-like experience.

Party Type: Make & Take 101

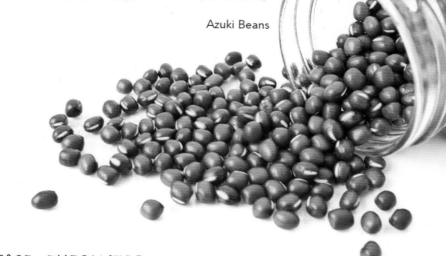
Azuki Beans

FACE EXFOLIATOR

Ingredient:
- 4 ounce Glass Jar
- Organic Raw Coconut Oil (Alternative: Sweet Almond Oil)
- ¼ cup Azuki Beans (dried and ground in a coffee grinder)
- Alternatives: Ground Almonds, Baking Soda, or Cane Sugar
- Distilled Water
- 20 drops Lemon and 10 drops Melrose™ Essential Oils
- PSK Alternative Essential Oils: 10 drops each Lemon, Lavender, and Frankincense

DIY Directions: Melt Coconut oil in a double boiler until just melted. Remove from heat immediately. Pour melted Coconut oil into glass bowl. Add essential oils and ground Azuki beans and blend well. Add some water to desired consistency. Scoop into jar.

Directions for Use: After face is fully cleansed, use a warm facecloth over your face for 15 seconds. Apply a small amount of Face Exfoliator in small circular motions. Rinse with warm water, then use a final rinse/splash of cool water to close up pores.

Party Type : Make & Take 102

EYE SERUM

Ingredients:
- 5mL Dropper Bottle
- Organic Raw Rosehip Seed and Jamaican Black Castor Oil
- 5 drops each Gentle Baby™, Sacred Frankincense, Myrrh, 3 drops each Sacred Sandalwood (optional) and Patchouli, 1 drop Rose (optional) Essential Oils
- PSK Alternative Essential Oils: 5 drops each Lavender, Frankincense, and Copaiba, 3 drops lemon

DIY Directions: Combine all essential oils in the dropper bottle. Swirl to blend. Add Jamaican Black Castor oil to about ½ full and fill to ¾ full with Rosehip Seed oil, leaving room for the dropper. Fasten the dropper cap on, then swirl the bottle to blend well.

Directions for Use: Apply 2-4 drops around eyes before bed. Gently pat around eyes. Do not get any directly into eyes. Not for use during the day if going into sunlight.
Party Type: Make & Take 102

FACE SERUM (ALL SKIN TYPES)

Ingredients:
- 10mL Dropper Bottle
- Organic Raw Grapeseed Oil
- 8-10 drops each of Lavender and Frankincense Essential Oils

DIY Directions: Combine Lavender and Frankincense in the dropper bottle. Swirl to blend the two oils. Add Grapeseed oil to about ¾ full, leaving room for the dropper. Fasten the dropper cap on, then swirl the bottle to blend well. This one is a customer favorite!

Directions for Use: Apply a dime-size amount (about 8 drops) all over freshly-washed face, neck, and back of hands both morning and night.

Party Type: Make & Take 101

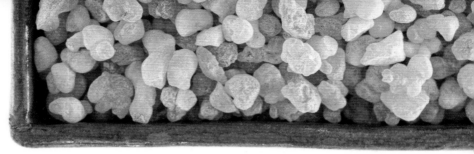

Frankincense Resin

FACE SERUM (BLEMISH SUPPORT)

Ingredients:
- 10mL Dropper Bottle
- Organic Raw Grapeseed Oil or Pumpkin Seed Oil
- 15 drops Melrose™ Essential Oil
- PSK Alternative Essential Oils: Purification® alone, or 5 drops each Lavender, Lemon, and Frankincense

DIY Directions: Fill Grapeseed or Pumpkin Seed oil to about ¾ full, leaving room for the dropper. Add Melrose™ essential oil blend. Fasten the cap on, then swirl the bottle to blend well.

Directions for Use: Apply a dime-size amount (about 8 drops) all over freshly-washed face, neck, or anywhere that is needed, morning and night.

Party Type: Make & Take 101

FACE TONER SPRAY

Ingredients:
- 4 ounce Glass Spray Bottle
- 3 ounces Distilled Water or Homemade Lavender Hydrosol
- 5 drops each Lavender, Sacred Frankincense, and Sacred Sandalwood essential oils
- PSK Alternative Essential Oils: 5 drops each Lavender and Frankincense

DIY Directions: Combine all essential oils into spray bottle and swirl around to blend. Add distilled water or hydrosol and shake to mix.

Directions for Use: Spray directly onto face morning and night or anytime as needed. Keep in the refrigerator for longer shelf-life. Use product within 1-2 weeks if not in the refrigerator, or up to 1 month if kept in the refrigerator.

Party Type: Make & Take 102

FINGERNAIL SUPPORT

Ingredients:
- 5mL Dropper Bottle
- Jojoba Oil
- 5 drops each Lemon, Lavender, Frankincense and Myrrh (optional) Essential Oils

DIY Directions: Combine the essential oils in the dropper bottle and swirl to blend. Add Jojoba oil and swirl to blend.

Directions for Use: Massage onto fingernails twice a day.

Party Type: Make & Take 101 or 102

FIZZIES (BATH BOMBS)

Ingredients:
- Glass Jar
- Flexible Mold
- 1 cup Citric Acid
- 1 cup Baking Soda
- 1 ½ cups Corn Starch
- 1-2 teaspoons Grapeseed Oil
- Plant Based Food Coloring
- Lavender Essential Oil

DIY Directions: Combine Citric Acid, Baking Soda, and Corn Starch. Slowly drizzle a small amount of Grapeseed oil into the mix, kneading until it feels like wet sand. Be careful not to add too much Grapeseed oil otherwise you may activate the Citric Acid and ruin the mix. Add a natural, plant-based coloring. Smooth into a flexible mold of your choice or plastic globe molds. Add 1-3 drops Lavender essential oil per mold depending on mold size. Let dry completely. Gently pop Fizzies out of molds and store in an airtight glass jar.

Directions for Use: Drop 1-2 Fizzies into your warm bath.

Party Type: Make & Take 102

FRAGRANCE

Ingredients :
- 5mL Fragrance Atomizer
- Witch Hazel
- Essential Oil Blend of Choice

  Create one of the following recipes:
    - 8 drops Tangerine Essential Oil and 2 drops Vanilla Absolute (Not Grocery Store Extract)
    - 6 drops Lemongrass, 4 drops Rosemary, and 2 drops Peppermint
    - PSK Alternative Essential Oil: 8 drops Stress Away™

DIY Directions: Combine the essential oils in the atomizer and swirl to blend. Add Witch Hazel and shake to mix well.

Directions for Use: Spray on pulse points as desired.

Party Type: Make & Take 102

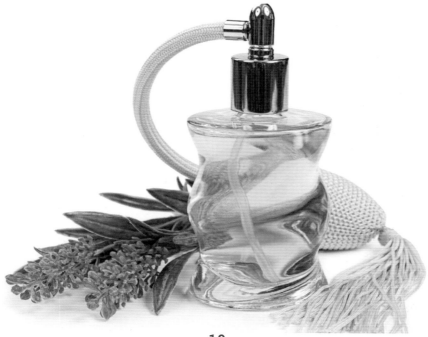

HAND LOTION

Ingredients:

- 4 ounce Glass Jar
- ¼ cup Shea Butter
- 2 tablespoons Sweet Almond Oil
- 1 tablespoon Beeswax (Vegan Alternative: Candelilla Wax)
- 20 drops Lime (for inside use only-omit Lime if in the sun), 10 drops each Lavender, Cedarwood, and Copaiba essential oils
- PSK Alternative Essential Oils: 20 drops Lemon (for inside use only-omit Lemon if going in the sun), 10 drops each Lavender, Copaiba, and Frankincense
- *NOTE: the citrus oils help brighten and even tone on the hands. If you go into the sun often, omit the citrus oils.*

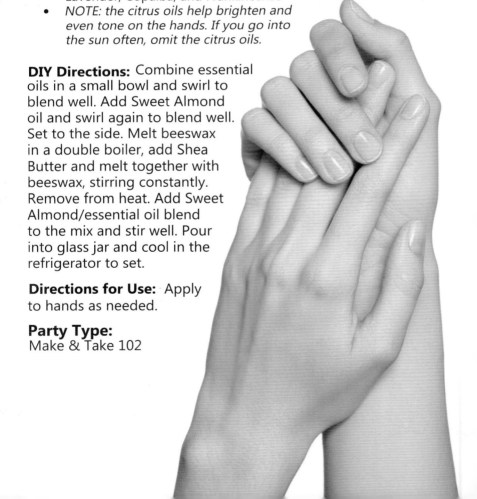

DIY Directions: Combine essential oils in a small bowl and swirl to blend well. Add Sweet Almond oil and swirl again to blend well. Set to the side. Melt beeswax in a double boiler, add Shea Butter and melt together with beeswax, stirring constantly. Remove from heat. Add Sweet Almond/essential oil blend to the mix and stir well. Pour into glass jar and cool in the refrigerator to set.

Directions for Use: Apply to hands as needed.

Party Type:
Make & Take 102

HAND SOAP (FOAMING)

Ingredients:
- 8 ounce Foaming Hand Soap Dispenser
- 6 ounces Distilled Water
- 2 tablespoons Liquid Castile Soap
- ¼ tablespoon Organic Sweet Almond Oil
- 10 drops Thieves® or Lavender Essential Oil

DIY Directions: Combine all ingredients into dispenser making sure to leave extra room for the pump.

Directions for Use: Pump some foam, and wash those hands!

Party Type: Make & Take 101

HAND SCRUBBING BALLS

Ingredients:
- Glass Jar
- Mini Globe Molds
- 1 cup Epsom Salt
- 1 cup Baking Soda
- ¼ cup Water
- 10-20 drops Lavender Essential Oil

DIY Directions: Grind Epsom Salt in a coffee grinder until it becomes a fine powder. Blend together with Baking Soda. Add 10-20 drops essential oil, then slowly mix in water until it becomes a stiff cookie dough consistency. Roll into small balls and place on wax paper or place into molds. Make balls about ¾ the size of the mold as the mix will expand as it dries. If using a mold, tape it shut or use a weight to keep it closed while it dries. Once fully dry, put balls into a glass container next to the sink.

Directions for Use: Use one ball to give your hands a good clean scrub.

Party Type: Make & Take 102

HAIR CONDITIONING RINSE

Ingredients :
- Large Glass Water Jug
- 1 cup Apple Cider Vinegar
- 1 cup Distilled Water
- 1 tablespoon Organic Honey (optional)
- 10 drops each Peppermint and Lavender, and 5 drops Rosemary (optional) Essential Oils

DIY Directions: Combine all essential oils into glass water jug and swirl to blend. Add honey and swirl to blend. Pour in Apple Cider Vinegar and swirl to blend again. Add distilled water and blend well.

Directions for Use: Apply to freshly-washed, damp hair and massage for 2 minutes. Rinse out completely, towel dry, and apply Hair Serum to the ends of hair. Style as usual.

Party Type: Make & Take 102

HAIR DEEP CLEANSER

Ingredients:
- 2 ounce Dropper Bottle
- 1.75 ounces Distilled Water
- 20 drops each Tea Tree, Lemon, and Rosemary Essential Oils
- PSK Alternative Essential Oils: 20 drops each lemon and Lavender, 10 drops Frankincense

DIY Directions: Combine all essential oils into dropper bottle and swirl to blend. Top off with distilled water and shake to mix.

Directions for Use: Place dropper bottle into a bowl of hot water to warm up for 2 minutes. Wet hair in a warm shower. Apply directly to scalp while mix is still warm and rub into scalp and hair. Leave on for a minimum of 2 minutes while in the shower or a maximum of 10 minutes with a shower cap on. Rinse well and apply conditioner of choice.

Party Type: Make & Take 102

HAIR DEEP CONDITIONER

Ingredients:
- 1 Ripe Avocado
- 2 tablespoons Organic Honey
- 1 tablespoon Jamaican Black Castor Oil
- 5 drops each Geranium, Lavender, and Sacred Sandalwood Essential Oils
- PSK Alternative Essential Oils: 5 drops each Lavender, Frankincense, and Copaiba

DIY Directions: Combine all essential oils into bowl and swirl around to blend. Mash avocado until completely smooth and creamy. Use blender if necessary. Add Jamaican Black Castor oil and continue to blend. Add essential oil blend and mix well. Use recipe right after you make it. This is for a single use.

Directions for Use: Apply the entire mix to damp hair and cover with a plastic cap. Leave on for 30-60 minutes. Rinse completely out and apply Hair Serum to the ends of hair. Style as usual.

Party Type: Make & Take 102

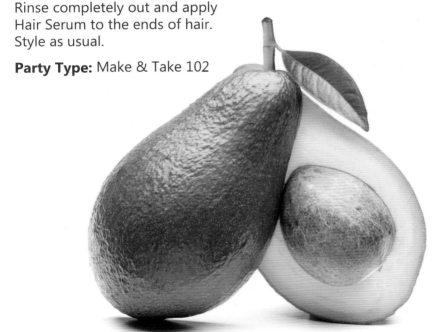

HAIR DETANGLING SPRAY

Ingredients:
- 4 ounce Glass Spray Bottle
- 2 ounces Distilled Water or Lavender Hydrosol
- 1 ½ teaspoons Apple Cider Vinegar
- 10 drops each Rosemary, Lavender, and Cedarwood Essential Oils
- PSK Alternative Essential Oils: 10 drops each Lavender, Copaiba, and Peppermint

DIY Directions: Combine all essential oils into the glass spray bottle and swirl to blend. (Optional: Wait 24 hours to allow oils to fully synergize.) Add 1.5 teaspoons of Apple Cider Vinegar. Shake bottle to fully blend ingredients. Add 2 ounces distilled water or Lavender hydrosol and shake again.

Directions for Use: Spray on dry or damp hair as needed. Shake gently before each use. Use entire spray within 2 weeks to maintain freshness of oils. Discard any unused portion after two weeks as oils may oxidize.

Party Type: Make & Take 102

HAIR DETANGLING SPRAY (EASY VERSION)

Ingredients:
- 4 ounce Glass Spray Bottle
- 3.5 ounces Distilled Water
- 1 tablespoon Copaiba Vanilla Conditioner

DIY Directions: Pour distilled water into glass spray bottle, add Copaiba Vanilla Conditioner and shake well.

Directions for Use: Spray on dry or damp hair as needed. Shake gently before each use. For added scent, consider adding 5 drops of Lavender essential oil.

Party Type: Make & Take 101

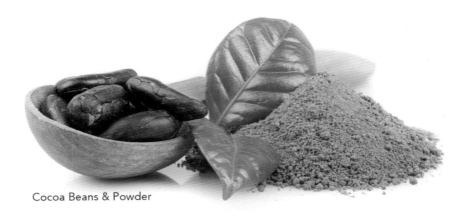
Cocoa Beans & Powder

HAIR DRY SHAMPOO

Ingredients:
- Empty Spice Shake
- ¼ cup Cornstarch (Alternative: Arrowroot)
- 1 tablespoon Baking Soda
- Optional for dark hair: 2 tablespoons Cocoa Powder
- 6 drops Lime, plus 3 drops each Tea Tree, Rosemary, Lavender and Cedarwood Essential Oils
- PSK Alternative Essential Oils: 6 drops Lemon, plus 3 drops each Lavender, Peppermint, and Copaiba

DIY Directions: Combine all essential oils into a clean bottle and swirl around to blend. Combine all dry ingredients into shaker container and shake to mix. Add essential oil blend and shake to mix.

Directions for Use: Sprinkle dry shampoo onto the roots of your hair and massage into your scalp. Leave on for 2 minutes, then shake out and brush through. To add shine back on ends, use hair Serum.

Party Type: Make & Take 102

HAIR FOLLICLE SPRAY

Ingredients:

- 4 ounce Glass Spray Bottle
- 3 ounces Distilled Water or Homemade Hydrosol using Lavender, Peppermint, or Rosemary (See Hydrosol recipe)
- *FOR WOMEN:* 20 drops each Peppermint, Lavender, Cedarwood, Rosemary, Cypress, Thyme, and Clary Sage Essential Oils
- *FOR MEN:* 20 drops each Peppermint, Lavender, Cedarwood, Rosemary, Cypress, Thyme, and Northern Lights Black Spruce Essential Oils
- PSK Alternative Essential Oils: 20 drops each Peppermint, Lavender, Frankincense, and Copaiba

DIY Directions: Combine all essential oils into spray bottle and swirl to blend. Add distilled water or hydrosol and shake to mix.

Directions for Use: Spray directly onto scalp morning and night . Keep in the refrigerator for longer shelf life. Use product within 1-2 weeks if not in the refrigerator, or up to one month if kept in the refrigerator.

Party Type: Make & Take 102

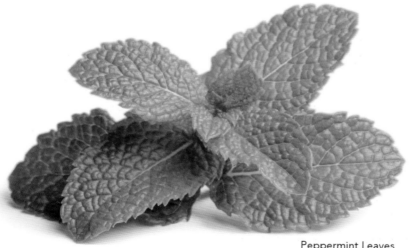

Peppermint Leaves

HAIR SERUM

Ingredients:

- 15mL Dropper Bottle
- Jojoba Oil or Grapeseed Oil
- 40 drops Jamaican Black Castor Oil
- 10 drops each Frankincense, Tea Tree, Rosemary, Lavender, Cedarwood, Clary Sage, and Lemon Essential Oils
- PSK Alternative Essential Oils: 10 drops each Frankincense, Lavender, Lemon, and Copaiba

DIY Directions: Combine all essential oils into a 15mL bottle and swirl to blend. Add 40 drops of Jamaican Black Castor oil and top off with Jojoba oil for coarse or wavy/curly hair or Grapeseed oil for straight or fine hair. Swirl bottle to blend.

Directions for Use: Use 2-5 drops. Rub hands together to warm up the oil and apply to the ends of hair first, working your way up to mid-shaft. Do not apply to roots or top of head. Use the small leftovers to gently pat down flyaway hairs.

Party Type: Make & Take 102

HAIR SHAMPOO

Ingredients:

- 8-16 ounce Hard Plastic or Glass Pump Bottle
- Distilled Water
- Castile Soap
- 20 drops Lavender and 10 drops Peppermint Essential Oils

DIY Directions: Combine essential oils into pump bottle and swirl to blend. Fill halfway with Castile soap and swirl to blend. Top off with distilled water and shake to mix.

Directions for Use: Pump a generous amount into hands and lather onto wet hair. Rinse and repeat if desired.

Note: If you have been using traditional shampoo, expect a transition period of up to 6 months while your hair and scalp adjust. During this period, it is important to use Hair Follicle Spray and Hair Serum on wash days, and as needed on in-between days. You can use Copaiba Vanilla Shampoo by Young Living to help with the transition period.

Party Type: Make & Take 102

HAIR SPLIT END SPRAY

Ingredients:
- 2-4 ounce Glass Spray Bottle
- 2 ounces Distilled Water or Lavender Hydrosol
- 1 teaspoon Jojoba Oil
- 10 drops each Frankincense, Rosemary, Lavender, Cedarwood, and Clary Sage Essential Oils
- PSK Alternative Essential Oils: 10 drops each Frankincense, Lavender, and Copaiba

DIY Directions: Combine all essential oils into the glass spray bottle and swirl to blend. Add 1 teaspoon of Joioba oil. Shake bottle to fully blend ingredients. Add 2 ounces distilled water and shake again.

Directions for Use: Spray on dry or damp hair as needed 1-2 times per day. Shake gently before each use. Use entire spray within 2 weeks to maintain freshness of oils. Discard any unused portion after two weeks as oils may oxidize.

Party Type: Make & Take 102

HAIR SHINE SPRAY

Ingredients:
- 2 ounce Glass Spray Bottle
- 2 ounces Distilled Water or Lavender Hydrosol.
- 10 drops each Sacred Sandalwood, Rosemary, Geranium, and Lavender Essential Oils
- PSK Alternative Essential Oils: 10 drops each Lavender and Copaiba

DIY Directions: Combine all essential oils into the glass spray bottle and swirl to blend. Add 2 ounces distilled water and shake to fully blend ingredients.

Directions for Use: Spray on dry or damp hair as needed 1-2 times per day. Shake gently before each use. Use entire spray within 2 weeks to maintain freshness of oils. Discard any unused portion after two weeks as oils may oxidize.

Party Type: Make & Take 102

HEEL AND FOOT CREAM

Ingredients:

- 4 ounce Glass Jar
- ¼ cup Shea Butter
- ¼ cup Raw Coconut Oil
- 2 tablespoons Beeswax (Vegan Alternative: Candelilla Wax)
- 10 drops Frankincense, 10 drops Lavender, 10 drops Bergamot, 5 drops Tea Tree, and 5 drops Oregano Essential Oils
- PSK Alternative Essential Oils: 10 drops each Frankincense, Lavender, Lemon, and Peppermint

DIY Directions: Combine the essential oils in the glass jar and swirl to blend. Place the lid on and set to the side. Melt Beeswax in a double boiler, add Shea Butter and melt together, stirring constantly. Remove from heat and add Coconut oil and mix well. While still liquid, pour contents into glass jar containing the essential oils. Place lid on tightly and shake to blend well. Place in refrigerator to set.

Directions for Use: Massage onto feet morning and night.

Party Type: Make & Take 102

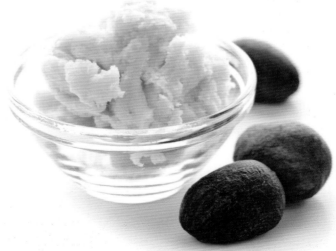

Shea Nuts & Butter

HOME: CANDLES (LAVENDER BUD)

Ingredients:

- 1-2 sheets Natural Beeswax (8" x 16" Natural Color)
- 1-2 feet Candle Wick
- 2 tablespoons Organic Lavender Buds
- 5-10 drops Lavender Essential Oil

DIY Directions: Working on a flat, clean surface, place one sheet of beeswax in front of you. Measure the short width of the sheet and cut candle wick to ½ inch longer than the short width. In a

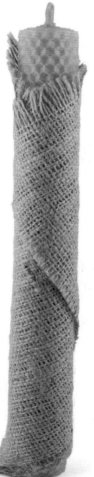

separate small bowl, wind up cut candle wick and drip 5-10 drops of Lavender essential oil to fully saturate the wick. Pull wick out and pour Lavender buds into bowl. Unwind wick and place straight along the very end of the short end of the beeswax sheet, leaving ½ inch of wick sticking over one end (this will be the top of your candle). Starting from one corner, fold over a very small part of the beeswax to wrap around the wick. Use a hairdryer to warm up the wax a bit to make it more pliable. Do not melt. Continue working up the wick, wrapping it with the edge of the beeswax. Once the entire wick is wrapped, start to roll the wick up in the beeswax like you would roll up a carpet. Keep the roll as tight as possible without smashing down the hexagon pattern too much. When there are 4 inches left on the roll, stop rolling and sprinkle Lavender Buds on the inside of the leftover 4 inches. Spread out evenly or make a pattern, making sure they are all flat on the beeswax while keeping the final ¼ inch edge free and clear. Gently pat them down. Continue to roll the candle. Once finished, smooth the final ¼ inch edge down using the warmth of your fingers to tack it down. Using glue, apply Lavender Buds to the outside bottom for decoration. Trim wick to ¼ inch. Tap down base edge to stand up.

Directions for Use: Create two candles and wrap with ribbon for a wonderful gift. Use as decoration in a bathroom, or light for a peaceful Lavender Candle experience. Remember to use a candle base to catch any wax drips.

Party Type: Make & Take 101 or 102

HOME: DEGREASER

Ingredients:
- Large Hard Plastic or Glass Spray Bottle
- 2 cups Distilled Water
- 1 cup White Vinegar
- 1 tablespoon Baking Soda
- 1 teaspoon Castile Soap
- 20 drops of Thieves® and 20 drops Orange Essential Oils
- PSK Alternative Essential Oils: 20 drops Thieves® and 20 drops lemon

DIY Directions: Combine all ingredients and shake to blend.

Directions for Use: Shake before each use. Spray liberally on surface and let sit for 5 minutes. Spray again to keep wet for a total of 15 minutes. Wipe clean .

Party Type: Make & Take 102

HOME: DRAWER SACHETS (LAVENDER)

Ingredients:
- 2 Quilting Squares (Zig-Zag Edged)
- Fabric Glue
- Small Funnel
- 2 tablespoons Organic Lavender Buds
- 5 drops Lavender and Cedarwood (optional) Essential Oils

DIY Directions: Place one quilting square with the outside facing down. Edge with fabric glue about 1/8 inch from the edge all the way around, leaving a 1 inch area unglued on one side. The glue will look like a boxy letter "C". Place second quilting square directly on top with outside facing up. Let fully dry. Place Lavender buds in a small bowl and infuse with Lavender and Cedarwood essential oils. Cover and shake to mix. Once quilting squares are fully dry, slide a funnel into the small opening on the side and fill with Lavender buds. Glue the opening shut and place a weight on it to keep tacked down. Once fully dry, shake sachet to activate the scent.

Directions for Use: Place Lavender Sachet into lingerie drawer or small space, such as a car or office drawer.

Party Type: Make & Take 101

HOME: ROOM FRESHENER

Ingredients:
- 4 ounce Glass Spray Bottle
- 2 ounces Distilled Water
- 2 ounces Witch Hazel
- 8-10 drops of Essential Oil of Choice

DIY Directions: Fill bottle with distilled water and Witch Hazel, then add essential oils and shake to blend. For a kid's room spritzer, use Stress Away™ for bedtime calming and decorate with a fun label for "Monster-Away Spray."

Directions for Use: Spray in the air as needed or directly onto pillows and fabric.

Party Type: Make & Take 101

HOME: WINDOW CLEANER

Ingredients:
- Large Hard Plastic or Glass Spray Bottle
- 2 cups Distilled Water
- ¼ cup White Vinegar
- ¼ cup Rubbing Alcohol
- 1 tablespoon Cornstarch
- 2 ounces Witch Hazel
- 10 drops of Thieves® and 10 drops Orange or Lemon Essential Oil

DIY Directions: Combine all ingredients into spray bottle and shake to blend.

Directions for Use: Shake well before each use. Spray on glass and surfaces for a streak-free shine. Use a microfiber cloth so there is no lint left on the windows.

Party Type: Make & Take 102

HYDROSOL

Ingredients:

- Fresh Organic Plants such as Peppermint, Lavender, or Rosemary. Make sure they are the correct Latin binomial. *Mentha piperita, Lavandula angustifolia, or Rosmarinus officinalis.*
- Large Stainless Steel Pot with Lid
- Small Ramekin
- Medium Bowl to fit on top of Ramekin inside the large pot
- Distilled Water
- Ice Cubes
- 2-4 ounce Glass Spray Bottle
- Suggested Essential Oils to Add: Lavender, Peppermint, Frankincense, and/or Copaiba

DIY Directions: Place ramekin upside down in large pot. Place medium bowl on top. There should be at least two inches of space around the entire pot area from the medium bowl outside edge to the large pot outside edge. Add cut up plants in the large pot at the bottom around the ramekin. Fill with distilled water to just cover the plants. Put on low heat. Do not allow water to boil. It should be hot enough to have steam but not boil. Place the large pot lid over the pot upside down so the lid handle is underneath. Place ice on the upside-down lid. As the steam rises, the ice will cool it causing it to create liquid condensation that will then drip down into the medium size bowl. This is the Hydrosol. Allow the water to collect for 20-30 minutes. Continue to add ice as needed to the upside-down lid. Pour Hydrosol into 4 ounce bottle and store in the refrigerator.

Directions for Use:

Add your favorite essential oils to your Hydrosol and label for use. Common uses are for hair and face sprays. Store in refrigerator for longer shelf life.

Party Type:

Make & take 102

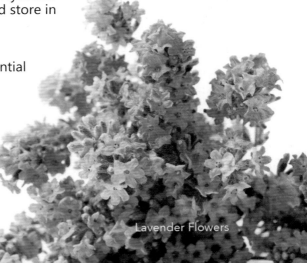

Lavender Flowers

LIP BALM

Makes: About 1 Dozen Tubes

Ingredients:
- 2 tablespoons Shea Butter
- 2 tablespoons Raw Coconut Oil (Alternative: Jojoba Oil)
- 1.5 tablespoons Beeswax Pellets. Use 2 TBSP for stiffer lip balm. (Vegan Alternative: Candelilla Wax)
- 30 drops Essential Oil (suggestions: Peppermint, Lavender, Grapefruit, or your favorite blend)

DIY Directions: On wax paper, line up tubes about 3 inches apart with caps off on a clear surface. Melt Shea Butter, Coconut oil, and Beeswax together in a double boiler. Stir constantly until fully melted. Turn off burner and add essential oils. Blend in well. While still warm and melted, use a pipette to fill lip balm tubes. Let tubes cool completely at room temperature before placing caps on.

Directions for Use: Apply to lips as needed!

Party Type: Make & Take 102

LIP SCRUB

Makes: About 6 Mini Containers

Ingredients:
- 3 teaspoons Brown Sugar
- 2 tablespoons Raw Coconut Oil (Alternative: Jojoba Oil)
- 1 teaspoon Molasses (Alternative: Organic Honey)
- 3 drops Lemon, 2 drops Ginger, 1 drop Nutmeg, 1 drop Cinnamon Bark Essential Oils
- PSK Alternative Essential Oils: 3 drops Lemon, 2 drops Thieves®

DIY Directions: Blend all essential oils in small clean bottle and swirl to blend. Set aside. In small bowl, blend Coconut oil, Brown Sugar, and Molasses until mixed well. Add essential oil blend. Scoop into mini jars.

Directions for Use: Apply small amount to lips and gently scrub in a circular motion. Wipe off excess to reveal smooth, soft lips.

Party Type: Make & Take 101

MAKEUP REMOVING PADS

Ingredients:
- 4 ounce Glass Jar (to fit cotton rounds)
- 24 Cotton Rounds
- ¼ cup Witch Hazel
- 2 tablespoons Sweet Almond Oil
- 2 tablespoons Distilled Water
- 2 teaspoons Castile Soap
- 5 drops each of Lavender and Frankincense Essential Oils

DIY Directions: Stack cotton rounds into the glass jar and set to the side. In a separate mixing bowl, add essential oils and swirl to blend. Add Sweet Almond oil and Castile soap and swirl to blend. Add both Witch Hazel and Distilled Water and blend well. Pour mix over the cotton rounds in the glass jar.

Directions for Use: Remove makeup with pads.

Party Type: Make & Take 101

LUCY LIBIDO'S "SKINAMINT"
(EDIBLE PERSONAL LUBRICANT) www.lucylibido.com

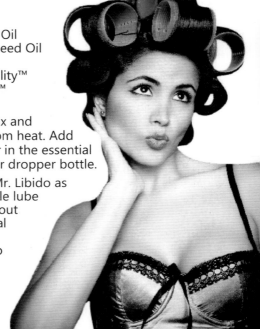

Ingredients:
- ½ teaspoon Beeswax
- 3 teaspoons Raw Coconut Oil
- 3 teaspoons Edible Grapeseed Oil
- ¼-½ teaspoon Agave
- 4-5 drops Peppermint Vitality™
- 8 drops Grapefruit Vitality™
- 2 drops Orange Vitality™

DIY Directions: Melt the Beeswax and Coconut oil together. Remove from heat. Add the Agave and Grapeseed oil. Stir in the essential oils. Store in a pump top bottle or dropper bottle.

Directions for Use: Named by Mr. Libido as tasting like "Skinamint", this edible lube will change the way you think about flavored lubes... no nasty chemical flavor, and it feels AHHH AHHH AHHmaaaazing on. It contains no preservatives, so check for freshness each time it's used.

Party Type: Make & Take 101

MANLY AFTERSHAVE

Ingredients:
- 15mL Dropper Bottle
- Witch Hazel
- 30 drops Aloe Vera Juice
- 5 drops each Myrrh, Frankincense, and Bergamot (*Young Living's is Furanocoumarin-free and will not cause a burn when in the sun*), Plus 10 drops Northern Lights Black Spruce Essential Oils
- PSK Alternative Essential Oils: 15 drops Thieves® or 5 drops each Frankincense, Peppermint, and Copaiba

DIY Directions: Combine essential oils in dropper bottle and swirl to blend. Add Aloe Vera juice and swirl to blend. Top off with Witch Hazel, place dropper cap on tightly, and shake to blend.

Directions for Use: Shake bottle before opening. Apply a small amount into the palm of your hand, rub hands together and pat all over freshly-shaved skin.

Party Type: Make & Take 102

MANLY BEARD BALM

Ingredients:
- 4 ounce Glass Jar
- 3 tablespoons Raw Coconut Oil or Sweet Almond Oil
- 2 tablespoons Shea Butter or Mango Butter
- 1-2 tablespoon Beeswax (based on desired stiffness, add more to make more stiff, less to make smoother)
- 10 drops Sacred Sandalwood, 6 drops Bergamot, 3 drops Clove Essential Oils
- PSK Alternative Essential Oils: 10 drops Frankincense, 6 drops Lemon, 3 drops Peppermint

DIY Directions: Cover a low heat double boiler, melt beeswax until just melted. Add Shea or Mango Butter and stir until melted. Add Coconut or Sweet Almond oil and continue to stir. Combine all essential oils into jar and swirl around to blend. Remove from heat and pour into jar with essential oils. Place lid on tightly and swirl to blend. Do not open until fully cooled and set.

Directions for Use: Scoop out a small amount, rub in hands to warm up, and apply to beard as usual. Store in a cool dry place.

Party Type: Make & Take 102

MANLY BEARD OIL

Ingredients:
- 10mL Dropper Bottle
- Jojoba Oil
- 9 drops Patchouli, 6 drops Bergamot, 4 drops Clove, 4 drops Rosemary, 3 drops Cedarwood, and 2 drops Lemongrass Essential Oils
- PSK Alternative Essential Oils: 10 drops Cobaiba, 5 drops Frankincense, 5 drops Lemon

DIY Directions: Combine essential oil in dropper bottle and swirl to blend. Top off with Jojoba oil and swirl to blend.

Directions for Use: Apply small amount to beard as needed.

Party Type: Make & Take 102

MANLY MUSCLE SUPPORT

Ingredients:
- 10mL Dropper Bottle
- Grapeseed Oil
- 20 drops each PanAway®, Peppermint, and Copaiba Essential Oils

DIY Directions: Combine essential oil in dropper bottle and swirl to blend. Top off with Grapeseed oil and swirl to blend.

Directions for Use: Apply to muscles before and after a workout.

Party Type: Make & Take 102

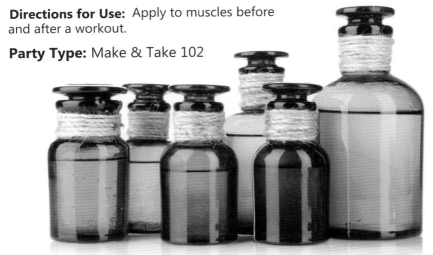

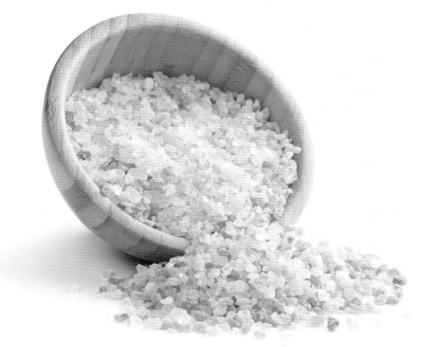

Pink Himalayan Sea Salt

MOUTHWASH

Ingredients:
- 8 ounce Glass Jar
- 1 cup Distilled Water
- 2 teaspoons Calcium Carbonate Powder (optional)
- ¼ teaspoon Pink Himalayan Sea Salt
- 10 drops Peppermint, 8 drops Thieves®, and 5 drops Lemon Essential Oils

DIY Directions: Blend all essential oils in small, clean bottle and swirl to blend. Set aside. In 8 ounce jar, add distilled water, Calcium Carbonate, and Pink Himalayan Sea Salt. Shake to mix. Add essential oil blend and shake to mix.

Directions for Use: Gargle morning and night with ½ ounce, then spit out for a fresh clean mouth.

Party Type: Make & Take 102

NIPPLE BUTTER (FOR NURSING MOMMY)

Ingredients :
- 4 ounce Glass Jar
- 3 tablespoons Raw Coconut Oil (Alternative: Jojoba Oil)
- 2 tablespoons Cocoa Butter
- 1.5 tablespoons Beeswax (Alternative: Candelilla Wax)
- 5 drops each Helichrysum, Geranium, Myrrh, Frankincense, and Lavender Essential Oils
- PSK Alternative Essential Oils: 10 drops each Frankincense and Lavender

DIY Directions: Combine essential oils in jar and swirl to blend. Melt Beeswax in a double boiler until just melted. Add Cocoa Butter and stir until melted. Turn off burner and add Coconut oil. Continue to stir until fully blended. Pour mix into jar containing essential oils. Place lid on and swirl jar to blend well.

Directions for Use: Apply to nipples as needed between nursing.

Party Type: Make & Take 102

POTTY-POURRI SPRAY

Ingredients:
- 4 ounce Glass Spray Bottle
- ¼ cup Witch Hazel
- 2 tablespoons Everclear® Grain Alcohol (190 Proof Vodka)
- 2 tablespoons Vegetable Glycerin
- 5-10 drops Blue Food Coloring (optional for visual effect)
- 30 drops Purification® Essential Oil

DIY Directions: Combine all ingredients in glass spray bottle. Shake vigorously to blend.

Directions for Use: Spray liberally onto toilet bowl water surface prior to use.

Party Type: Make & Take 102

ROLLERBALLS

Ingredients:
- 5mL Rollerball
- Organic Raw Grapeseed Oil
- 8-12 drops Essential Oil Recipe of Choice

Create one of the Following combos:
- Sleep/Focus Support: Stress Away™
- Critter Control: Purification®
- Shoulder/Foot Massage: PanAway®
- Breathe Support: 4 drops each Lavender, Lemon, and Peppermint
- Easy Pre-Mixed Blends: Simply pump directly from one of the Young Living Massage Oils and fill up the 5mL Rollerball. Use Sensation™, OrthoSport ™, or OrthoEase™ without any additional carrier oil.

DIY Directions: Add essential oils to the 5mL rollerball and top off with Grapeseed oil.

Directions for Use:
- **Sleep/Focus Support Roller:** Apply to the back of the neck, along the spine, on the wrists, or on the big toes.
- **Critter Control Roller:** Apply all over the bottom of the feet and along the hairline.
- **Shoulder/Foot Massage Roller**: Apply over the shoulder area or feet and massage in.
- **Breathe Support Roller:** Apply on the skull behind the ears and down both jawlines.

Party Type:
Make & Take 101

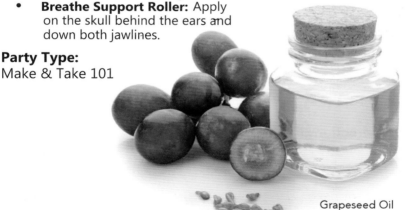

Grapeseed Oil

SCALP SERUM MASK

Ingredients:
- 15mL Dropper Bottle
- Jamaican Black Castor Oil
- 10 drops each of any three or five of the following essential oils: Peppermint, Tea Tree, Frankincense, Lavender, Cedarwood, Rosemary, Clary Sage, Thyme, Cypress, Northern Lights Black Spruce, Peppermint, Lemon, or Orange
- PSK Alternative Essential Oils: 10 drops each Peppermint, Lavender, Frankincense, Lemon, and Copaiba

DIY Directions: Combine essential oils into dropper bottle and swirl around to blend. Top off with Jamaican Black Castor oil and swirl to blend. This is for a single use.

Directions for Use: In a small bowl filled with hot water, place dropper bottle with top tightly in place into bowl. Let warm up for 2 minutes. Wet hair with hot water and apply warm serum all over your scalp. Use any left over to pull through the ends of hair. Tie up in a bun if you have long hair. Place shower cap over entire head and let set for 10-30 minutes. Wash thoroughly with sulfate-free shampoo.

Party Type:
Make & Take 102

SCALP SPRAY (FLAKE SUPPORT)

Ingredients:
- 4 ounce Glass Spray Bottle
- 3 ounces Distilled Water
- 10 drops each Peppermint, Lavender, Tea Tree, and Rosemary, Essential Oils
- PSK Alternative Essential Oils: 10 drops each Peppermint, Lavender, and Frankincense

DIY Directions: Combine all essential oils into spray bottle and swirl to blend. Add distilled water and shake to mix.

Directions for Use: Spray directly onto scalp twice per day.

Party Type: Make & Take 102

SUNSCREEN (SPF 35)

Ingredients:
- 4 ounce Glass Jar
- 2 tablespoons Cocoa Butter
- 1 tablespoon Beeswax (Vegan Alternative: Candelilla Wax)
- ½ tablespoon Carrot Seed Oil *(Note: Carrot Seed Oil is not the same as Carrot Essential Oil-There is no SPF in any essential oil.)*
- ½ tablespoon Red Raspberry Seed Oil
- 1 tablespoon Zinc Oxide Powder (Non Nano)
- 10 drops each Lavender and Frankincense Essential Oils

DIY Directions: In a double boiler, melt Cocoa Butter until melted. Turn off burner and add Carrot Seed and Red Raspberry Seed oils and blend well. Add essential oils and stir well. Slowly stir in Zinc Oxide powder while covering mouth and nose with a mask. Add a small amount at a time until it is fully blended into lotion. Use an electric mixer for several minutes to evenly distribute ingredients. Pour lotion into jar and seal tightly to let cool.

> *Note: Zinc Oxide powder is very fine. Wear gloves and mask and do not allow any to get into your lungs. Do not have small children in the room when working with Zinc Oxide. While Zinc Oxide is a natural ingredient and is non-toxic, it should not be inhaled.*

Directions for Use: Apply to exposed skin while in the sun. This sunscreen is water-resistant but not waterproof. Reapply after swimming or every 30 minutes (depending on skin burn rate) if in the water all day. Reapply every 1-2 hours or as needed.

Party Type:
Make & Take 102

TOENAIL SUPPORT

Ingredients:
* 5mL Dropper Bottle
* Jojoba Oil
* 10 drops each Lavender, Oregano, and Tea Tree Essential Oils
* PSK Alternative Essential Oil: 20 drops each Thieves® and Lavender

DIY Directions: Combine the essential oils in the dropper bottle and swirl to blend. Add Jojoba oil and swirl to blend.

Directions for Use: Massage onto toenails twice per day.

Party Type: Make & Take 101

TOOTH POLISH

Ingredients:
* 2 ounce Glass Jar or Tube
* 4 tablespoons Baking Soda
* 1 tablespoon Raw Coconut Oil (Alternative: Grapeseed Oil)
* 10 drops Thieves® and 10 drops Peppermint essential Oils

DIY Directions: Blend all essential oils in small clean bottle and swirl to blend. Set aside. In small bowl, blend Coconut oil and Baking Soda until mixed well. Add more or less baking soda to desired consistency. Add essential oil blend. Scoop into mini jars.

Directions for Use: Apply a pea-size amount to toothbrush. Gently brush upper teeth in a downward pulling motion from the top of your gums to the bottom of your teeth, and for your lower teeth going upward from the base of your gums up through the tips of your teeth. Brush your tongue, then spit out excess. You may rinse or leave small leftovers in mouth.

Party Type: Make & Take 101

UNDERARM SUPPORT

Ingredients:
- 3 tablespoons Baking Soda
- 3 tablespoons Coconut Oil (Alternative: Jojoba Oil)
- 2 tablespoons Shea Butter (Alternative: Cocoa Butter)
- 1 tablespoon Cornstarch (Alternative: Arrowroot)
- 1 tablespoon Beeswax (Vegan Alternative: Candelilla Wax)
- 1 tablespoon Sweet Almond Oil (Alternative: Grapeseed or Rosehip Seed Oil)
- 20 drops Purification® and 10 drops each Lavender and Cypress essential oils
- PSK Alternative Essential Oils: 20 drops Purification® and 10 drops Lavender

DIY Directions: Combine Shea Butter, Beeswax and Coconut oil in a double boiler until melted. Turn off burner. Combine Baking Soda and Cornstarch then add to mix and stir well. Add Sweet Almond oil and essential oils and blend well. Pour into containers. Let cool fully.

Directions for Use: Rub onto armpits.
Note: If you have never used natural deodorant, you should expect a transition period. To help support additional detox odor, use one drop of Purification® neat on armpits before you rub on Underarm Support. Detox can last 2-6 weeks.

party type: Make & Take 102

UNDERARM SUPPORT (EASY)

Ingredients:
- 5mL Rollerball
- Jojoba or Grapeseed Oil
- 20 drops Purification® Essential Oil

DIY Directions: Add essential oil to rollerball and top off with Grapeseed oil.

Directions for Use: Roll onto armpits.

Party Type: Make & Take 101

WHIPPED BODY BUTTER

Ingredients :
- 2 ounce Glass Jar
- ½ cup Shea Butter
- ½ cup Raw Coconut Oil (Alternative: Jojoba Oil)
- ½ cup Sweet Almond Oil (Alternative: Grapeseed Oil)
- 1 teaspoon Vitamin E Oil
- 15 drops of your favorite Essential Oil, such as Lavender, Peppermint, or Stress Away™

DIY Directions: Melt Shea Butter in a double boiler. Add Coconut and Sweet Almond oil and melt together, stirring constantly. Remove from heat and cool in the refrigerator for an hour to slightly set without getting hard. Remove from refrigerator, and using a hand mixer, blend well until you obtain a whipped consistency. Add essential oils to final whipping stage. Scoop into glass jar.

Directions for Use: Apply as needed.

Party Type: Make & Take 102

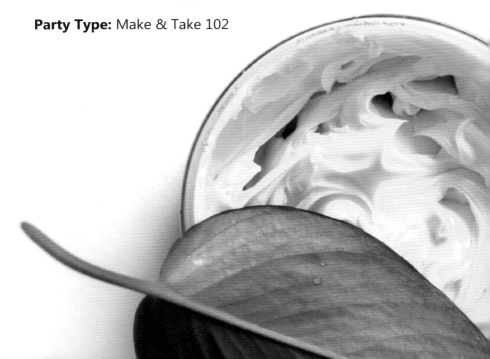

FINAL THOUGHTS

It can be very empowering to make your own products and be 100 percent confident of your ingredients. It's even better that your products have ingredients that you can actually read and pronounce . (Jojoba oil is pronounced *Hohoba*, in case you wondered.) I am a busy mom who really just wants to hang out with my family. I limit any and all extra busy work in my life as much as possible. So when it comes to making my own products, I want them to be quick and easy.

This book contains my quick, easy, and sometimes dirty recipes ('cuz let's be real, I am a mess in the kitchen) that are so much healthier for me and my family — plus, most are pennies on the dollar from what I would have spent at the store. Okay, so the *Whipped Body Butter* takes a little more time and energy, so, for that reason, it is only in my house about once a year. You know, the time of year I start to feel like" Suzy Homemaker" and I get the gumption to go on a hunt for my hand mixer. I'm usually hoping to find BOTH beaters, but I've been known to make use of just one in a pinch.

The reality is we are all busy, but our health should not take a back seat. I always say, "When mom is down, we all are down." Somehow my house just seems to completely disintegrate when I am not well. These chemical-free products will help eliminate the majority of the endocrine disruptors in your life. Did you catch that!? Endocrine disruptors! They are all around you, even *right now* as you read this.

What are endocrine disruptors? First let's understand what your endocrine system is. Your endocrine system is the engine for your entire hormonal system. Your hormones are like your soil. If a plant's soil is depleted and bad, the whole plant looks terrible and produces nothing. So if your endocrine system is being disrupted, YOU will look terrible and YOU will produce nothing. Yikes!

Now, moving on to those sneaky little disruptors. I said they are all around you and I am not joking. Not even a little bit. The ink on this very page you are reading is a synthetic and could cause a disruption to your endocrine system if you are around publishing ink enough. (Rest assured, as a reader of books you are fine, but if you worked in a print house, you could experience some hormone issues long term.) Here are just a few to demonstrate the insidiousness of these disruptors.

KNOWN ENDOCRINE DISRUPTORS

Household cleaners, pharmaceuticals, phytoestrogens found in soy, bovine protein, household dust (huge), plastic storage containers... plus, there are many hidden endocrine disruptors found in just about everything from kids' toys to nail polish, antiperspirants, shampoos and conditioners with parabens and sulfates, body wash, toothpaste, lotions, sunscreens, shaving gel, cosmetics, plastic bottles that contain BPA, Teflon® pans and baking molds, tampons, laundry detergent, dryer sheets, fabric softeners, dishwasher detergent, mattresses, memory foam, fire retardants, air fresheners, synthetic fragrances, vinyl shower curtains, electric blankets, anti-bacterial hand soap containing triclosan, insect repellent, phthalates found in so many things it is scary: fragrances, shampoo, air fresheners, new car smell, steering wheel, vinyl flooring—the list goes on and on! You can see a full list of chemicals to avoid at www.ewg.org or the EWG app.

What's a girl to do? Go back through this book and earmark every single page with the recipes you need to make! They are really not that hard, and you can start replacing all of your chemically yuckiness one product at a time. Consider this: if you simply tackled one recipe per week, you could replace over 50 items in your house in a year! They each only take around 10 minutes or less to make, so time is not an excuse. You can slowly build up your supply base by purchasing ingredients here and there and then use them throughout the year, so money is also not an excuse (except for the *Sunscreen*, that is a bit pricey but WAY worth the chemical crap storm you are avoiding from store-bought brands). Remember, these products will actually SAVE you money. Here are some comparisons of my own savings.

Dove® Deodorant	$4.39	vs. $1.50
Tom's® Toothpaste	$3.99	vs. $2.80
Neutrogena® Toner	$7.49	vs. $2.40
Neutrogena® Makeup Remover	$6.49	vs. $2.60
Neutrogena® Moisturizer	$9.99	vs. $5.80
Neutrogena® Eye Cream	$17.99	vs. $6.50
Paul Mitchell® Smoothing	$20.99	vs. $8.90
Windex®	$3.14	vs. $2.10
Febreze® Air Effects	$5.09	vs. $1.70
Beard Guyz™ Beard Balm	$14.99	vs. $6.40
Bourdeaux's® Paste	$7.99	vs. $2.50
	$102.54	**$43.20**

THAT'S A SAVINGS OF $59.34! Um , yes please!

I hope you are empowered and energized to clean up your home and lifestyle! Reach out to the person who gave you this book and make things together! Get a group of ladies to go in together to split the costs on bulk items to make it even more inexpensive and fun. Enjoy this journey, and I wish you all the success for a more happy and healthful life!

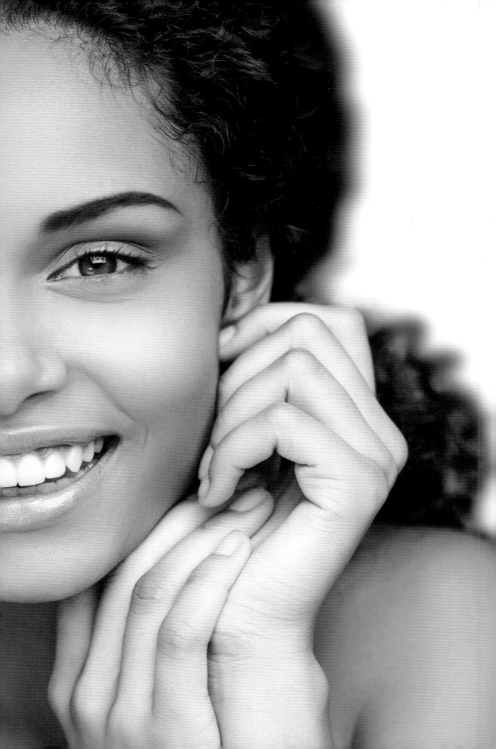

RESOURCES

Brands:
- Cocojojo
- Dr. Adorable
- Dr. Bronner's
- Liquid Gold
- Mary Tyler Naturals
- Natural Way Organics

Retailers:
- Amazon
- eBay
- Life Science Publishing
- My Oily Habit
- New Directions Aromatics
- Trader Joe's

EQUIPMENT LIST

- Coffee Grinder
- Electric Mixer
- Funnel
- Measuring Cups
- Measuring Spoons
- Mixing Bowl
- Molds
- Pipettes
- Pyrex Bowls
- Ramekin, Small
- Stainless Steel Pot
- Large Lid

SUPPLY LIST

Obtain glass when available.

- Atomizer, Fragrance
- Candle Wick
- Containers, Small
- Cotton Rounds
- Dropper Bottles
- Fabric Glue
- Foaming Soap Dispenser
- Jars, Glass
- Pump Bottle
- Quilting Squares
- Rollerballs
- Spice Shaker
- Spray Bottle, Glass
- Tubes, Lip Balm Size
- Tubes, Deodorant size
- Water Jug, Glass

INGREDIENT LIST

- Almonds, ground
- Aloe Vera Gel
- Aloe Vera Juice
- Apple Cider Vinegar
- Arrowroot
- Avocado
- Azuki Beans
- Baking Soda (Not Baking Powder)
- Beeswax Pellets
- Beeswax Sheets
- Brown Sugar
- Calcium Carbonate Powder
- Candelilla Wax
- Cane Sugar
- Carrot Seed Oil
- Castile Soap-Dr. Bronner's
- Castile Soap-Natural Way Organics
- Citric Acid
- Copaiba Vanilla Conditioner (Young Living)
- Cocoa Butter
- Cocoa Powder (Unsweetened)
- Coconut Oil (Organic,raw)
- Cornstarch
- Distilled Water
- Egg White
- Essential Oils (Young Living)
- Everclear® Grain Alcohol (190 Proof Vodka)
- Food Coloring
- Grapeseed Oil
- Honey (Organic)
- Jamaican Black Castor Oil
- Jojoba Oil
- Lavender Buds (Organic)
- Mango Butter
- Massage Oils (Young Living)
- Molasses
- Oats, Gluten Free (Quick Oats)
- Pumpkin Seed Oil
- Sweet Almond Oil

- Red Raspberry Oil
- Rosehip Seed Oil
- Rubbing Alcohol
- Salt — Dead Sea
- Salt — Epsom
- Salt — Pink Himalayan
- Saponified Coconut Oil Liquid Soap
- Shea Butter
- Sugar — Brown
- Sugar — Cane, Raw
- Vegetable Glycerin
- Vitamin E 0il
- White Sugar
- White Vinegar
- Witch Hazel
- Zinc Oxide Powder

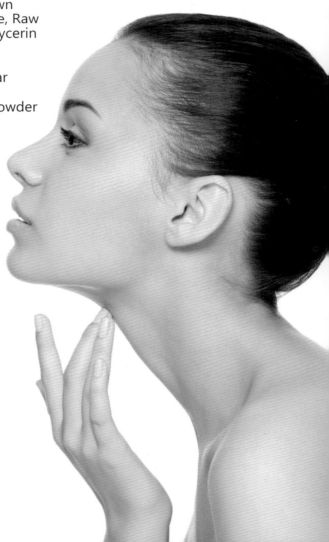

ADDITIONAL EDUCATION

BOOKS

- "The Essential Oil Truth: The Facts Without The Hype" by Jen O'Sullivan
- "French Aromatherapy: Essential Oil Recipes & Usage Guide" by Jen O'Sullivan
- "Essentially Driven: Young Living Essential Oils® Business Handbook" by Jen O'Sullivan
- "Gameplan: The Complete Strategy Guide to go from Starter Kit to Silver" by Sarah Harnisch
- "Lucy Libido Says.....There's an Oil for THAT: A Girlfriend's Guide to Using Essential Oils Between the Sheets" by Lucy Libido
- "Essential Oil Desk Reference" 7th Edition, Life Science Publishing
- "Healing Oils of the Bible" by Dr. David Stewart
- "Essential Oils Integrative Medical Guide" by D. Gary Young, ND
- "D. Gary Young: The World Leader in Essential Oils" by Mary Young

EDUCATION

- The EO Bar App
- Facebook.com/groups/TheHumanBody
- Facebook.com/groups/IgniteAcademy
- Instagram.com/theEObar
- The School for Aromatic Studies

  Free Introduction to Essential Oils:
  www.courses.aromaticstudies.com/product/introduction-to-aromatherapy/

  Essential Wellness:
  www.courses.aromaticstudies.com/essential-wellness/

  French Foundations:
  www.courses.aromaticstudies.com/certificate-in-french-aromatic-foundations/

EDUCATIONAL TOOLS

www.31oils.com
Educational books, essential oil usage brochures, new member starter challenge cards, essential rewards explanation cards, company comparison charts, and more.

AUTHOR BIOGRAPHY

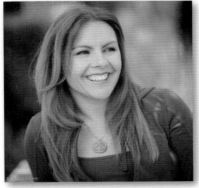

Jen O'Sullivan is the author of multiple best-selling books on aromatherapy and is certified in French Medicinal Aromatherapy through The School for Aromatic Studies. She has been a professional educator since 1999, at both the collegiate and high school levels. She is lovingly known as "The oil lady to the oil ladies" and has the ability to take complicated information and share it in a way that makes it easy to understand. Jen lives in Southern California with her husband and High School sweetheart, Tim and their son, Jacob. She is an avid Bible scholar and Jesus follower, cyclist, mountain biker and snowboarder, professional-turned-hobbyist photographer, gluten-free health nut yet totally addicted to sugar, copious reader, stay-at-home mom, devoted wife, and general lover of life.

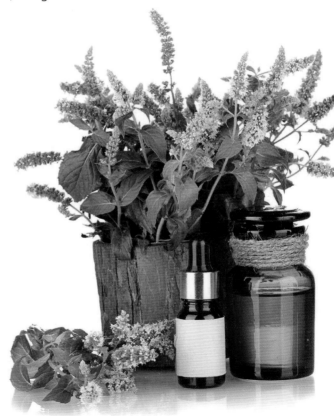

Made in the USA
Middletown,DE
17 May 2017